GASTROPARESIS MANAGEMENT DIET COOKBOOK

Delicious Recipes For Improved Digestion And Wellness Healing: Rich Dishes For Managing Digestive Challenges

DR. SHAYLA LEWIS

Table of Contents

CHAPTER ONE 14
  Gastroparesis: What is it? 14
    Typical Signs and Causes 14
      Diet is Crucial for Managing Gastroparesis 15
    The gastroparesis management diet is based on the following important ideas: 16
    Low-Fiber Foods: 16
  Low-Fat Options: 17
    Fluid Intake 17
    How to Begin the Diet for Gastroparesis Management: 18
    Creating Reasonable Objectives: 18
      Essential Kitchen Items for Simple Meal Preparation: 19
    Advice for Meal Planning and Grocery Shopping 20
  The Value of Maintaining Hydration 21
    Including Exercise in Your Daily Routine: 21
    Getting Around the Foundations of Gastromatous Management 22

Comprehending the Diet for Gastroplasty: 23

Low-carbohydrate Foods 23

Foods High in Antioxidants: 23

Anti-inflammatory Foods: 24

CHAPTER TWO 26

The Value of Mindful Eating and Portion Control: 26

Maintaining Stable Blood Sugar Levels by Balancing Macronutrients: 26

Foods to Eat and Bad Foods to Avoid: 27

How to Modify Recipes to Meet Your Dietary Requirements: 28

Energising Morning Meals 30

Easy and Healthy Breakfast Ideas: 31

Smoothie Recipes for Easy Digestion: .32

Innovative Muesli Concoctions 32

Strategies for Handling Morning Nausea: 33

CHAPTER THREE 34

Filling Snacks and Starters: 34

Easy and Healthful Snack Ideas 35

Hummus and vegetable sticks: 36

Hard-boiled eggs: 36
Smoothies: 36
Trail mix: 37
Avocado and rice cakes 37
   Whole grain wraps with turkey and veggies: 37
Energy bars: 37
   Snacks high in nutrients to control blood sugar levels: 38
Nutrient-dense foods that help control blood sugar levels include: 38
Edamame: 39
Greek yogurt with granola: 39
Avocado hummus: 40
White bean dip: 40
Pumpkin seed pesto: 40
Roasted red pepper dip: 40
Smoothies: 41
Cooked vegetables: 42
   Advice for controlling hunger in between meals: 42
Make a plan 42
Eat nutrient-dense foods: 43

Keep yourself hydrated: 43
CHAPTER FOUR 44
Healthy Salads and Soups 44
Healthy Soups for Any Occasion 44
How to Make Your Own Homemade Broth 45
Adding Healthy Fats and Protein to Salads 46
Dressing Recipes: 47
scrumptious main courses 48
Cooking Methods 48
Selection of Ingredients: 49
Sample Cookbooks: 49
Optimal Dinner Ideas: 50
The composition of the plate 50
When to Eat: 51
Turkey and Vegetable Stir-Fry 51
Sources of Protein: 52
Cooking Techniques: 53
CHAPTER FIVE 54
Sample Cookbooks 54
Turkey Meatballs in Marinara Sauce: 54

Black Bean and Quinoa Stuffed Peppers: 54

Low-Carb Substitutes for Customary Favourites: 54

Replacements for Ingredients: 55

Changes to the Recipe: 55

Cauliflower Crust Pizza: 56

Eggplant Lasagna: 56

Turkey and Vegetable Lettuce Wraps: 56

One-Pot Dinner Ideas for Simple Cleanup 56

Cooking Methods: 57

Adaptable Substances: 57

Sample Cookbooks: 57

Lentil and Vegetable Soup: 58

Shrimp and Asparagus Risotto: 58

Adding Vegetables to Main Courses: .. 58

Innovative Cooking Techniques: 59

Inspiration for a Recipe: 59

Sample Cookbooks 60

Roasted Vegetable Quinoa Bowl: 60

Spinach & Mushroom Frittata: 60

Advice for Mindful Eating and Portion Control at Dinner: 60

Size of Portion: 61

Eating Conscientiously: 61

CHAPTER SIX 62

Paying Attention to Your Body: 62

Examples of Strategies 62

Delicious Side Dishes: 63

Delicious Side Dishes to Round Out Your Dinner: 63

Easy Ways to Include Legumes and Grains: 64

Innovative Ways to Prepare Vegetables: 65

How to Add Flavour Without Using Too Much Sugar or Fat: 65

Techniques for Reducing the Portion of Side Dishes: 66

Desserts and Sweet Treats: 67

Desserts That Are Both Rich and Nutritious 67

Recipes for sugarless desserts: 68

Desserts made with fruit for a naturally sweet taste: 69

Advice on how to sate desires without sacrificing your health objectives: 69

Techniques for regulating dessert portion sizes: 70

Smoothies and Beverages: 71

CHAPTER SEVEN 72

Ideas for Refreshing and Hydrating Drinks: 72

Smoothie Recipes Packed with Nutrients: 72

Components: 73

The Value of Maintaining Hydration . 74

Innovative Methods for Naturally Flavouring Water: 75

Social Events and Eating Out: 76

Investigate Restaurants in Advance: .. 76

Communicate Clearly with Servers: ... 77

Be Ready to Adjust Meals: 77

Emphasis on Easy Preparations: 78

Control Your Portion: 78

How to Effectively Communicate Your Dietary Needs: 78

Offer Suggestions: 79

Express Your Gratitude: 79

Make a Plan: 80

Eat Before You Go: 80

Emphasis on Socialising: 80

Bring Your Own Snacks: 81

CHAPTER EIGHT 82

Making Nutritious Decisions When Dining Out 82

Remain Hydrated: 82

Listen to Your Body: 82

Be Aware of Portion Sizes: ...83

Ideas for Organising Events That Are Gastroparesis-Friendly: 83

Urge Guests to Bring food: ...84

Upkeep and Extended Success: ...85

Maintaining Your Progress in Gastroparesis Management 85

Techniques for maintaining accountability and motivation 87

Advice for overcoming obstacles along the route 87

Rejoicing your accomplishments and maintaining an optimistic outlook: 88

THE END 96

© 2024 Dr. Shayla Lewis All rights reserved.

No part of this publication may be reproduced, distributed, or transmitted in any form or by any means, including photocopying, recording, or other electronic or mechanical methods, without the prior written permission of the publisher, except in the case of brief quotations embodied in critical reviews and certain other noncommercial uses permitted by copyright law.

DISCLAIMER

Write a brief complete Disclaimer for my diet cook book telling them that the author is not in any association with any company, business or individual and also this book is written by the authors knowledge and understanding

The information provided in this diet cookbook is based on the author's personal knowledge and understanding. The author is not affiliated with, endorsed by, or associated with any company, business, or individual. The recipes and dietary advice contained within this book are intended for informational purposes only. Readers should consult with a healthcare professional or a registered dietitian before making any significant changes to their diet or lifestyle. The author assumes no responsibility for any adverse effects that may result from the use or misuse of the information contained in this book.

CHAPTER ONE
Gastroparesis: What is it?

A gastrointestinal condition called gastroparesis is characterized by a delayed, mechanically unobstructed emptying of the stomach contents into the small intestine. It happens when the muscles or nerves that govern the stomach muscles malfunction. For those who have the illness, this delay in emptying can cause a number of symptoms and problems that lower their quality of life overall.

Typical Signs and Causes

Gastroparesis symptoms might differ from person to person, however, they frequently include bloating, vomiting, early satiety, nausea, abdominal pain, and blood sugar swings. If treatment is not received, these symptoms may increase over time and have a major influence on day-to-day activities.

Gastroparesis can be brought on by a number of illnesses, such as diabetes, autoimmune disorders, Parkinson's disease, neurological conditions, certain drugs, and prior stomach or intestinal surgery.

Diet is Crucial for Managing Gastroparesis

Diet is essential for improving digestion and controlling the symptoms of gastroparesis. It's critical to select foods that are easier to digest and move through the stomach more quickly because prolonged gastric emptying can worsen symptoms. This usually entails eating smaller, more often meals that are made up of easier-to-digest low-fat, low-fiber foods.

An overview of the benefits of this cookbook

The goal of this cookbook is to offer tasty and useful recipes that are especially suited for those who have gastroparesis. Through an emphasis on products and cooking techniques that facilitate simpler digestion and reduce symptoms, this cookbook is a useful tool for anyone managing the difficulties associated with having gastroparesis.

Essential Elements of the Diet for Gastroparesis Management

The gastroparesis management diet is based on the following important ideas:

Small, Frequent Meals: To avoid overfeeding the stomach and promote better digestion, people are advised to consume multiple smaller meals throughout the day as opposed to three large ones.

Low-Fiber Foods: Foods high in fiber can be harder to digest and make gastroparesis symptoms worse. As a result, low-fiber foods including cooked fruits and vegetables, white bread, and refined grains are frequently included in the diet.

Low-Fat Options: Eating foods high in fat might cause the symptoms of gastroparesis to worsen and delay stomach emptying. Choosing low-fat and oily foods, staying away from fried foods, and selecting lean protein sources can all help control symptoms.

Foods that are Soft and Easily Chewable: Foods with a soft texture and ease of chewing are easier for the stomach to break down and digest.

Fluid Intake: Maintaining enough hydration is critical for digestive health and general well-being. To avoid filling the stomach too much and making symptoms worse, it's crucial to keep an eye on how much fluid you're consuming.

People with gastroparesis can better manage their illness and enjoy tasty, satisfying meals without aggravating their symptoms by following these guidelines and trying out the dishes in this cookbook.

How to Begin the Diet for Gastroparesis Management:

A precise meal plan is necessary for people with gastroparesis, a disorder marked by delayed stomach emptying, in order to reduce symptoms and enhance quality of life. To guarantee adherence and success while starting a gastroparesis treatment diet, practical goals must be defined. Start by being aware of your unique dietary requirements, constraints, and preferences. Speak with a nutritionist or medical expert who specializes in managing gastroparesis to develop a customized strategy that meets your individual needs.

Creating Reasonable Objectives:

Long-term gastroparesis management success requires setting realistic goals. These objectives must be attainable, quantifiable, and long-lasting. First, decide which dietary adjustments or routines you wish to put into place. Some examples include eating less high-fat or high-fiber foods, consuming more easily digested foods, or switching to smaller, more frequent meals. To prevent overcommitting, make these adjustments to your schedule gradually. As you acclimatize to your new eating habits, remember to acknowledge and appreciate your little accomplishments along the road.

Essential Kitchen Items for Simple Meal Preparation:

Having the proper supplies and equipment in your kitchen might help you prepare meals more quickly and adhere to your gastroparesis management diet. Invest in basic kitchen appliances like a slow cooker to make soft, easily digested meals, a blender or food processor for pureeing foods, and portion-controlled storage containers for leftovers.

Stock your cupboard with essentials that are good for people with gastroparesis, such as low-fiber grains (white rice, pasta), canned fruits and vegetables (seed and skin removed), lean meats (fish, poultry), and low-fat dairy products.

Advice for Meal Planning and Grocery Shopping:

Meal preparation and efficient grocery shopping are essential for managing gastroparesis. When you go grocery shopping, make sure to get complete, fresh meals that are easier to digest and reduce symptoms. Select refined grains, lean meats, and fruits and vegetables that are low in fiber. Carefully read food labels to steer clear of high-fiber or high-fat substances that may aggravate symptoms. To avoid stuffing your stomach, during meal planning, try to have smaller, more frequent meals and snacks throughout the day. To satisfy your dietary needs, create meals that are nutrient-dense and well-balanced, using a range of food groups.

The Value of Maintaining Hydration

For general health and wellbeing, especially in those with gastroparesis, enough water is crucial. Drinking enough water can aid in better digestion, reduce bloating and pain, and prevent constipation. Make it a goal to stay hydrated throughout the day by selecting hydrating drinks such as herbal tea, clear broth, and water. Steer clear of fizzy or caffeinated drinks as some people may find that they exacerbate their symptoms. Drink water gradually in between meals to avoid feeling queasy or excessively full.

Including Exercise in Your Daily Routine:

For those with gastroparesis, regular exercise can have a number of advantages, such as better digestion, stress reduction, and weight management. To support gastrointestinal motility and general well-being, include mild activity in your daily routine, such as yoga, swimming, or walking. Choose enjoyable and tolerable activities by paying attention to your body. As your fitness level increases, start out slowly and then increase the duration and intensity of your workouts. Before beginning any new fitness program, speak with your doctor, particularly if you have any underlying medical concerns.

Getting Around the Foundations of Gastromatous Management:

A comprehensive approach to care is necessary to alleviate symptoms and enhance general well-being in individuals with gastroparesis, a condition marked by delayed stomach emptying. Understanding the Gastroparesis Diet, which consists of a variety of foods and eating practices designed to facilitate digestion and reduce discomfort, is essential to this care.

Comprehending the Diet for Gastroplasty: The Gastroparesis Diet focuses on choosing meals that are less taxing on the stomach by being simpler to digest. Choosing foods that are anti-inflammatory, high in antioxidants, and low in carbs is a fundamental principle.

Low-carbohydrate Foods: Because they digest more slowly, carbohydrates might be difficult for people with gastroparesis to consume. Low-carb foods are better since they are easier on the stomach and less likely to exacerbate symptoms like bloating and nausea. Examples of these foods are leafy greens, non-starchy vegetables, and lean proteins.

Foods High in Antioxidants: Common symptoms of gastroparesis include inflammation and oxidative stress, both of which antioxidants are vital in preventing. A range of antioxidants that support gastrointestinal health can be obtained by including fruits and vegetables such as bell peppers, kale, and spinach, as well as citrus fruits and berries.

Anti-inflammatory Foods: It's critical to incorporate anti-inflammatory foods in the diet since chronic inflammation can aggravate the symptoms of gastroparesis. This includes foods high in green tea, turmeric, ginger, and omega-3 fatty acids—found in fatty fish like salmon and flaxseeds—all of which have strong anti-inflammatory qualities.

CHAPTER TWO

The Value of Mindful Eating and Portion Control:

In order to control food intake and reduce discomfort, portion control and mindful eating are essential components of gastroparesis care. By avoiding overfeeding the digestive system with smaller, more frequent meals throughout the day, symptoms like bloating and fullness can be minimized. Eating mindfully improves digestion and nutrient absorption by focusing on hunger and satiety cues, digesting food well, and enjoying every meal.

Maintaining Stable Blood Sugar Levels by Balancing Macronutrients:

For those who have gastroparesis, it is critical to keep blood sugar levels steady because variations can exacerbate symptoms and have an adverse effect on general health. This stability can be attained by balancing the macronutrients—fats, proteins, and carbohydrates—in each meal. By consuming complex carbohydrates with lean proteins and healthy fats, you can reduce the rate at which glucose is absorbed and avoid blood sugar spikes and crashes.

Foods to Eat and Bad Foods to Avoid:
Foods that aggravate the symptoms of gastroparesis should be avoided or eaten in moderation. Foods heavy in fat, fried foods, spicy foods, caffeine, alcohol, and carbonated drinks are some examples of these, as they can all cause discomfort by delaying the emptying of the stomach. On the other hand, foods like cooked vegetables, lean meats, whole grains, and low-acid fruits are better for those with gastroparesis since they are easier to digest and less harsh on the stomach.

How to Modify Recipes to Meet Your Dietary Requirements:

It takes ingenuity and inventiveness to modify recipes to fit the dietary constraints linked to gastroparesis.

The following advice can be used to alter recipes

Use healthier substitutes for high-fat foods, such as Greek yogurt in place of sour cream or olive oil in place of butter.

Instead of frying or grilling, choose cooking techniques that are easier on the stomach, such as steaming, baking, or poaching.

Play around with low-acid sauces, herbs, and spices to improve flavor without aggravating symptoms.

To increase digestion, reduce the amount of fibrous substances or purée them.

Watch portion sizes and try not to overeat because heavier meals might strain the digestive tract.

Through comprehension of the fundamentals of the Gastropteresis Diet and the application of techniques for mindful eating and recipe adjustment, people can efficiently handle their illness and enhance their standard of living.

Breakfast Delights: For those who are managing gastroparesis in particular, breakfast is frequently seen as the most significant meal of the day. It establishes the tone for your day's energy and digestion.

The goal of "Breakfast Delights" in a Gastroparesis Management Diet Cookbook is to offer enticing morning dishes that are nourishing and pleasurable but also easy on the stomach.

This section contains a selection of recipes that have been thoughtfully created to meet the unique dietary requirements of people who have gastroparesis. Every recipe, whether they are inventive variations on comfort food favorites or nourishing meals, is meant to promote healthy digestion.

Energising Morning Meals: The book "Energising Morning Meals" concentrates on offering breakfast choices that will both jump-start your day and provide you long-lasting vitality. It's critical for people with gastroparesis to eat foods that are both easily digested and high in nutrients to keep their bodies functioning.

The recipes in this section focus on using items that will not upset your stomach and will provide you a quick energy boost to get through the day. There is something here to satisfy every taste while meeting your nutritional requirements, whether you favor savory or sweet foods.

Easy and Healthy Breakfast Ideas: This section focuses on making things simple without sacrificing nutrition. It provides nutrient-dense but simple-to-make breakfast options that need no preparation. These recipes, which range from scrambled tofu to quick muesli bowls, are ideal for hectic mornings when time is of importance.

Including Fibre and Protein in Your Meal: Especially for those who are coping with gastroparesis, fiber, and protein are essential parts of a well-balanced meal. They assist in sustaining good digestion, promoting fullness, and stabilizing blood sugar levels.

The recipes in this section concentrate on adding foods high in protein and fiber to breakfast dishes without overburdening the digestive system. These dishes offer inventive methods to increase protein and fiber intake, from blending beans into savory breakfast bowls to adding nut butter to smoothies.

Smoothie Recipes for Easy Digestion: Smoothies are a great choice for those who have gastroparesis since they are simple to make and can be tailored to meet certain dietary requirements. Many smoothie recipes that are gentle enough not to irritate digestive ailments can be found in this section.

These smoothie recipes, which range from fruity blends to creamy creations, are meant to assist optimal digestion while offering a wholesome and revitalizing start to your day.

Innovative Muesli Concoctions: Muesli is a morning mainstay, renowned for its nourishing and cosy qualities. You'll find inventive muesli recipes in this section that go beyond the classic bowl of oats.

Some recipes offer creative takes on a traditional morning dish, such as savory muesli with veggies or sweet options like apple cinnamon muesli. Every version is made to meet the specific dietary requirements of people with gastroparesis while still offering vital nutrients.

Strategies for Handling Morning Nausea: Those suffering from gastroparesis may frequently experience morning nausea, which can make it difficult to eat breakfast. This section offers helpful advice and techniques for properly treating morning sickness.

These suggestions, which range from dietary adjustments to lifestyle adjustments, are meant to help people minimize discomfort and get a good start to the day. These tips, which include rearranging meal schedules and including anti-nausea foods, can help alleviate morning sickness and improve general health.

CHAPTER THREE

Filling Snacks and Starters:

It might be difficult to locate enjoyable snacks and appetizers that are also easy on the stomach when you have gastroparesis. To promote general health and well-being, it is crucial to make sure that these smaller meals offer enough nourishment.

Using easily digestible and pleasantly palatable ingredients is one way to create delicious snacks and appetizers. Choosing nutrient-dense foods in modest portions can assist supply the energy and nutrients required without taxing the digestive system.

Lean proteins, good fats, and complex carbs are a few components that can be used to make appetizers and snacks that are filling and beneficial to digestive health. Furthermore, adding herbs and spices can improve flavor without making the stomach feel bloated.

Easy and Healthful Snack Ideas:

Having easy access to quick and healthful snack options is crucial for people experiencing gastroparesis. These snacks ought to be simple to make, light on the stomach, and full of the vital nutrients that promote general health.

For managing gastroparesis, a few quick and healthful food options are as follows:

Greek yogurt with almonds and honey: Greek yogurt has a high protein content that can help with blood sugar stabilization and satiety. Extra taste and texture can be added by sprinkling in almonds and drizzling in honey.

Nut butter on whole grain crackers: Nut butter, such as peanut or almond butter, offers protein and healthy fats; whole grain crackers, on the other hand, give fiber and complex carbs.

Hummus and vegetable sticks: A delicious and wholesome snack can be created by combining crunchy veggies like carrots, cucumbers, and bell peppers with creamy hummus.

Hard-boiled eggs: Eggs are a convenient snack option and a rich source of protein that can be prepared in advance.

Smoothies: A nutrient-dense, easily digested snack can be made by blending fruits, vegetables, and protein-rich components like Greek yogurt or protein powder.

Ideas for portable snacks to eat while moving:

It is essential to have portable snack options on hand for controlling gastroparesis when traveling. Having easy-to-eat snacks on hand might help you stay full and avoid hunger throughout the day, whether you're traveling or just out and about.

Here are some suggestions for portable snacks to help manage gastroparesis:

Trail mix: This portable and nutrient-dense food alternative is made up of a mixture of nuts, seeds, and dried fruits.

Avocado and rice cakes: Avocado adds fiber and good fats, while rice cakes are light and simple to digest.

Whole grain wraps with turkey and veggies: These easy and filling wraps are made with whole grain tortillas, sliced turkey, and veggies like cucumbers, tomatoes, and lettuce.

Nut butter packets on an individual basis: Nut butter packets on an individual basis offer a source of protein and healthy fats and are perfect for on-the-go eating.

Energy bars: Seek for bars composed of simple, quickly digested components like almonds, dried fruits, and oats.

Snacks high in nutrients to control blood sugar levels:

For people with gastroparesis, it's critical to keep blood sugar levels steady in order to minimize energy surges and crashes and to keep symptoms from getting worse. A balanced intake of carbohydrates, protein, and healthy fats from nutrient-dense snacks can help maintain blood sugar levels all day.

Nutrient-dense foods that help control blood sugar levels include:

Almond butter with apple slices: Almond butter has healthy fats and protein, while apples have fiber and carbohydrates that help control blood sugar levels.

Berries and cottage cheese go well together since the former is high in protein and the latter offers fiber and antioxidants that help control blood sugar.

Edamame: Edamame beans are a great option for regulating blood sugar levels because they are a strong source of fiber and protein.

Greek yogurt with granola: the former supplies protein, while the latter supplies carbohydrates for long-term energy.

Chia seed pudding: Packed with fiber and omega-3 fatty acids, chia seeds make this nutrient-dense snack a great way to keep blood sugar levels stable.

Appetizing recipes for spreads and dips:

Spreads and dips can offer vital nutrients to appetizers and snacks while enhancing flavor and variety. Selecting dishes that are easy on the stomach and produced with easily digested ingredients is crucial while managing gastroparesis.

Avocado hummus: Tahini, garlic, lemon juice, chickpeas, and avocado combine to make a tasty, creamy dip that is easy on the stomach.

Greek yogurt, cucumber, garlic, and dill combine to make a light and delicious dip called tzatziki. It goes great with whole-grain crackers or veggie sticks.

White bean dip: This creamy, smooth, high-protein, and high-fiber dip is made with white beans, olive oil, lemon juice, and herbs.

Pumpkin seed pesto: This bright and fragrant pesto, which can be spread over crackers or sandwiches, is made with pumpkin seeds, basil, garlic, olive oil, and lemon juice.

Roasted red pepper dip: A tasty, nutrient-dense dip that is easy on the stomach and is made with roasted red peppers, almonds, garlic, and olive oil.

Adding fruits and vegetables to snack foods:

A balanced diet must include fruits and vegetables since they are rich sources of vitamins, minerals, and antioxidants. Choosing fruits and vegetables that are soothing on the stomach and easy to digest is crucial while managing gastroparesis.

Adding fruits and vegetables to snacks can help treat gastroparesis in a number of ways.

Smoothies: For a nutrient-dense and easily digested snack, blend fruits like bananas, cherries, and mangoes with leafy greens like kale or spinach.

Carrots, cucumbers, and bell peppers are some examples of chopped vegetables that are served with a mild dip or spread, like hummus or yogurt tzatziki.

Fruit salad is a light and delicious food that is easy on the stomach. Diced fruits such as melon, grapes, and kiwi should be combined.

Cooked vegetables: For an easy and wholesome snack, steam or roast veggies like sweet potatoes, squash, and zucchini until they are soft.

Fruit smoothie bowls: To add texture and taste to a thick fruit smoothie, top it with sliced fruits, nuts, and seeds.

Advice for controlling hunger in between meals:

For those with gastroparesis, controlling appetite in between meals is crucial to preventing overindulgence or pain. Throughout the day, incorporating modest, nutrient-dense snacks can help sustain energy levels and ward off extreme hunger.

Here are some pointers to control your hunger in between meals:

Make a plan: Give yourself enough time to think over and prepare snacks in advance so that you will always have wholesome options on hand when hunger strikes.

To avoid experiencing extreme hunger later on, learn to listen to your body's signals of hunger and fullness. Snacking should be done as soon as you start to feel hungry.

Eat nutrient-dense foods: To help stabilize blood sugar levels and sustain energy levels, choose snacks that offer a combination of healthy fats, protein, and carbs.

Keep yourself hydrated: Sipping lots of water during the day will help sate your appetite and prevent you from feeling peckish in between meals.

Eat mindfully by taking your time, enjoying your snacks, and paying attention to the flavors and sensations while you eat. This will help you avoid overindulging.

CHAPTER FOUR

Healthy Salads and Soups

A gastroparesis management diet should start with soups and salads since they provide a solid balance of nutrients and mild flavors that are gentler on the digestive tract. Including hearty soups and salads in your diet can maximize comfort while reducing pain, whether you're craving cool crispness or cozy warmth.

Healthy Soups for Any Occasion

It's critical to adjust your diet to the changing seasons while making sure that your meals continue to be light on the stomach when controlling gastroparesis. Rich soups are adaptable and may be made to fit any season, offering warmth and nourishment all year round. There is a soup recipe to fit every taste and nutritional requirement, from light summertime broths with fresh herbs to hearty wintertime vegetable stews.

Simple-to-Comb Soup Recipes

When choosing foods, digestibility is crucial for those who have gastroparesis. Simple-to-digest soup recipes reduce discomfort and improve nutrient absorption because they are easy on the stomach. Lean proteins, low-fat broths, and cooked veggies are common ingredients in these dishes since they are easier for the stomach to process and digest.

How to Make Your Own Homemade Broth
A homemade broth provides rich flavor and vital nutrients without the additives and preservatives found in store-bought variants,

making it a staple of many soups that are suitable for people with gastroparesis.

To get the most flavor out of your homemade broth, choose lean cuts of pork, chicken, or fish and boil them with aromatic vegetables and herbs. You may further improve the broth's digestibility by straining it before using it, which will guarantee a calming and filling foundation for your soups.

scrumptious salad combos

Any diet for managing gastroparesis would benefit from the refreshing inclusion of salads, which offer vital vitamins, minerals, and fiber in a light, readily digestible form. A range of tastes and textures, such as juicy fruits and creamy cheeses, crisp greens, and crunchy vegetables, are combined to create tasty salad combinations. You may make salads that are delicious and easy on the stomach by carefully choosing your ingredients and avoiding too hot or acidic ones.

Adding Healthy Fats and Protein to Salads

For those with gastroparesis, protein and healthy fats are vital nutrients that maintain general health and provide long-lasting energy. By adding these nutrients to salads, you may improve the taste and texture of your food while also promoting satiety and blood sugar balance. Salads can be enhanced with lean proteins, like grilled chicken or tofu, and healthy fat sources, like avocado or almonds, to make filling and wholesome meals.

Dressing Recipes: Enhance Flavour Without Getting Inflamed

Salads can benefit greatly from the flavor and moisture that dressings bring to them without bothering the digestive tract. Making your own dressings gives you more control over the ingredients and helps you stay away from typical triggers like vinegar and citrus, which can make your gastroparesis symptoms worse. Rather, go for light dressings consisting of olive oil, lemon juice, herbs, and spices. These sauces add flavor without being overpowering or causing upset stomachs. You can find dressings that both promote the health of your digestive system and your taste preferences by experimenting with different ingredient combinations.

scrumptious main courses

A key component of diet-based gastroparesis management is consuming tasty main dishes. Making food that is both scrumptious and easy on the stomach is a problem. One strategy is to concentrate on cooking techniques that bring out the flavor without using a lot of fat or spices that could aggravate symptoms.

Cooking Methods:

Tougher meat slices can be made more palatable by braising or slow cooking.

Roasting or grilling veggies can enhance their inherent sweetness and give a meal more flavor.

Herbs and mild spices, such as turmeric and ginger, can add flavor without upsetting the stomach.

Selection of Ingredients:

Lean proteins digest more easily than fatty meats, so choose to consume fish, chicken, and tofu instead.

Select seasonal, fresh products to enhance flavor and nutritional content.

Try using whole grains as the foundation for your main courses, such as brown rice or quinoa, which provide fiber and complex carbohydrates that will keep you full for longer.

Sample Cookbooks:

Lemon Herb Baked Chicken: Baked till golden brown, tender chicken breasts are marinated in a mixture of lemon juice, garlic, and fresh herbs.

Grilled Salmon with Dill Sauce: Perfectly cooked fresh salmon fillets are served with roasted asparagus and a mild dill yogurt sauce.

Tofu Stir-Fry with Mixed Vegetables: Savoury ginger soy sauce is used to sauté tofu cubes with vibrant bell peppers, broccoli, and snap peas.

Optimal Dinner Ideas:

For the purpose of managing gastroparesis, supper options that are balanced should include protein, carbs, and healthy fats in the right amounts to support sustained energy and digestive comfort.

The composition of the plate

Non-starchy vegetables, which are high in fiber, vitamins, and minerals, such as leafy greens, peppers, and cucumbers, should make up half of your plate.

Set aside a quarter of your plate for lean protein options, which include beans, fish, and grilled chicken. These foods include the critical amino acids needed for both satiety and muscle repair.

To supply complex carbs for energy, the remaining quarter can be made up of nutritious grains or starchy vegetables like quinoa or sweet potatoes.

When to Eat:

Distribute meals uniformly throughout the day to avoid packing the stomach and encourage easier digestion.

Steer clear of large, high-fat meals right before bed because they might aggravate GERD and other sleep-related issues.

Examples of Menus

Grilled Vegetable Quinoa Salad: Cooked quinoa, bell peppers, and cherry tomatoes are combined with a lemon vinaigrette to create a vibrant medley.

Turkey and Vegetable Stir-Fry: Brown rice is paired with lean ground turkey, broccoli, carrots, and snow peas sautéed in a garlic-ginger sauce.

Hearty Lentil Soup with Mixed Greens: Flavoured with cumin and coriander, this lentil soup simmers with kale, spinach, and carrots.

Recipes for Main Courses High in Protein:

Since it promotes general health and helps preserve muscle strength, protein is a crucial component for the management of gastroparesis. Including high-protein main course recipes in your diet will help you feel fuller between meals and supply the building blocks needed for tissue repair.

Sources of Protein:

Select lean meats that are easier to digest and have less fat, including skinless chicken breasts, turkeys, or pork loin.

Tofu, tempeh, beans, and lentils are plant-based proteins that can be included to create a vegetarian dish that is high in antioxidants and fiber.

Add fatty fish to your diet, including trout, salmon, or mackerel, which are rich in omega-fatty acids that are good for your heart and brain.

Cooking Techniques:
Baking, broiling, or grilling proteins can help them keep their flavor and moisture content without adding excessive fat.

Without depending on heavy sauces or spices, meats can be tenderized and given depth of flavor by marinating them in marinades made of yogurt or citrus juice.

CHAPTER FIVE

Sample Cookbooks

Turkey Meatballs in Marinara Sauce: Serve tender turkey meatballs over whole wheat spaghetti, cooked in a homemade marinara sauce flavored with Italian herbs and spices.

Black Bean and Quinoa Stuffed Peppers: Baked until golden, bell peppers are filled with cooked quinoa, black beans, corn, and diced tomatoes. Melted cheese is then placed on top.

Tofu Cubes marinated in a zesty peanut sauce, skewered with vibrant vegetables, and cooked to perfection are the ingredients of Grilled Tofu Skewers with Peanut Sauce.

Low-Carb Substitutes for Customary Favourites:

Low-carb substitutes for classic favorites can help reduce symptoms like bloating and pain while still satiating appetites for comfort foods that are familiar to those with gastroparesis.

Replacements for Ingredients:

To lessen the amount of carbohydrates and boost fiber, replace refined grains like white bread, spaghetti, and rice with whole grain alternatives like whole wheat bread, brown rice, or cauliflower rice.

For a lighter, more gastrointestinal-friendly choice, swap out high-carb components like potatoes or wheat-based goods with lower-carb substitutes like cauliflower, zucchini, or almond flour.

Changes to the Recipe:

Modify traditional recipes to cut back on processed foods and added sugars while increasing the amount of veggies and lean proteins.

Try using spiralized veggies, such as sweet potatoes or zucchini, in place of pasta in recipes like pad Thai or spaghetti carbonara.

Sample Cookbooks:

Cauliflower Crust Pizza: For a filling, low-carb supper, top a gluten-free pizza crust made of cauliflower, eggs, and cheese with tomato sauce, vegetables, and lean protein.

Eggplant Lasagna: For a cozy, low-carb take on a traditional meal, thinly slice eggplant and top it with marinara sauce, ricotta cheese, and spinach. Bake until bubbling and golden.

Turkey and Vegetable Lettuce Wraps: A tasty and light take on conventional wraps, this dish combines ground turkey with onions, peppers, and mushrooms, seasoned with Asian spices, and served in crisp lettuce leaves.

One-Pot Dinner Ideas for Simple Cleanup:

Not only are one-pot meal ideas quick and easy to prepare on hectic weeknights, but they also reduce mess and speed up the cooking process, which makes them perfect for people with gastroparesis.

Cooking Methods:

Cook several items at once in a pot or pan by using techniques like simmering, steaming, or stir-frying to maximize flavor and reduce the need for additional fats or sauces.

Select recipes that don't require a lot of chopping or preparation to ease the strain on the digestive system and simplify mealtimes.

Adaptable Substances:

To expedite meal preparation and cut down on cooking time, use adaptable foods like frozen veggies, canned beans, and precooked grains or proteins.

Use aromatics, such as onions, garlic, and ginger, to improve digestion and provide flavor without adding too much seasoning.

Sample Cookbooks:

Chicken and Vegetable Stir-Fry: Cooked brown rice or quinoa is paired with sliced chicken breast sautéed with colorful bell peppers, broccoli, and snap peas in a flavorful ginger soy sauce.

Lentil and Vegetable Soup: A filling one-pot supper that's high in protein and fiber, this hearty lentil soup is cooked with carrots, celery, and tomatoes while seasoned with herbs and spices.

Shrimp and Asparagus Risotto:

This luscious yet easily digestible supper option consists of creamy risotto prepared with soft shrimp, asparagus, and shallots, topped with a dusting of Parmesan cheese.

Adding Vegetables to Main Courses:
Including veggies in your major meals is a terrific way to increase their nutritional value. It also gives your meals more flavor, texture, and color, which makes them more aesthetically pleasing and enjoyable.

Innovative Cooking Techniques:
Try varied cooking techniques, such as grilling, roasting, or sautéing, to bring out the sweetness and caramelization of vegetables naturally rather than using a lot of seasonings or sauces.

Combine veggies with different textures and hues to create mouthwatering recipes that are visually appealing and gratifying to the senses.

Inspiration for a Recipe:

Add bulk and fiber to main meals like stuffed peppers, vegetable lasagna, or cauliflower crust pizza by using vegetables as the base or filling; this will cut down on the requirement for higher-calorie components.

To add extra nutrition and flavor to sauces, soups, or stews without sacrificing flavor or texture, blend veggies.

Sample Cookbooks

Roasted Vegetable Quinoa Bowl: A vibrant combination of cooked quinoa, and roasted veggies (including sweet potatoes, carrots, and Brussels sprouts), with a creamy tahini sauce.

Spinach & Mushroom Frittata: **For a delicious yet light supper, bake a fluffy egg frittata stuffed with sautéed spinach, mushrooms, and onions until brown. Serve with a side of mixed greens.**

Ratatouille with Herbed Couscous: A filling and healthy supper alternative, this traditional French meal consists of stewed tomatoes, eggplant, zucchini, and bell peppers served over herbed couscous.

Advice for Mindful Eating and Portion Control at Dinner:

When it comes to managing symptoms and enhancing overall digestive health, people with gastroparesis can benefit from mindful eating practices and portion control.

Size of Portion:

Reduce the size of your dishes and bowls to help you manage portion sizes and avoid overindulging.

To have a balanced meal, try to consume half of your plate with non-starchy veggies, 1/4 with lean protein, and 1/4 with whole grains or starchy vegetables.

Eating Conscientiously:

Give food enough time to be completely chewed, and enjoy every bite by focusing on the flavors, textures, and sensations that your mouth produces.

When eating, turn off devices like televisions and cellphones to concentrate on the meal and pay attention to your body's signals of hunger and fullness.

CHAPTER SIX

Paying Attention to Your Body:

To avoid pain or digestive problems, eat until you're content rather than stuffed, and stop when you feel comfortably full.

Be mindful of how different foods affect you and modify your diet accordingly. Keep a look out for any triggers or intolerances that can make symptoms worse.

Examples of Strategies

Before meals, engage in mindful breathing exercises or meditation to help calm the body and mind and improve digestion.

Maintain a food journal to record meals, serving sizes, and symptoms so that you can spot trends and choose your diet with knowledge.

You can enjoy delicious and satisfying meals while supporting digestive health and overall well-being by incorporating flavorful main courses, balanced dinner ideas, protein-rich recipes, low-carb alternatives, one-pot meal ideas, vegetable-centric dishes, and mindful eating strategies into your gastroparesis management plan.

Delicious Side Dishes: Improving Your Diet for Gastroparesis Management

Every meal decision matters while controlling gastroparesis, and side dishes are essential to completing a plate that is balanced. Let's be creative in creating delicious side dishes that satisfy the palate while adhering to the dietary restrictions that come with gastroparesis.

Delicious Side Dishes to Round Out Your Dinner:

Recipes for Healthy Side Dishes:

Your gastroparesis management diet cookbook's recipes, which highlight nutrient-dense foods like fruits, vegetables, whole grains, and lean proteins, are meant to fuel your body while easing digestive discomfort.

For tasty, simple-to-digest side dishes, try dishes like steamed broccoli with a lemon-garlic sauce, quinoa salad with cucumber and herbs, or roasted sweet potatoes.

Easy Ways to Include Legumes and Grains: Legumes and grains have stiff outer layers that might be problematic for people with gastroparesis, but they are also great sources of important minerals and fiber. For simpler digestion, choose well-cooked, softer varieties such as lentils, brown rice, or quinoa. You may even want to purée them.

To add these healthy elements to your diet without overburdening your digestive system, try trying meals like velvety mashed cauliflower with cannellini beans or a mild barley and vegetable soup.

Innovative Ways to Prepare Vegetables: Although vegetables are an essential part of any healthy diet, the fibrous texture of vegetables can make symptoms of gastroparesis worse. Use inventive cooking methods to soften and improve the flavor of vegetables, such as roasting, steaming, or sautéing.

For tasty, nutrient-dense side dishes that are gastroparesis-friendly, try recipes like stir-fried bell peppers and snap peas, steamed asparagus with lemon zest, or roasted root vegetables with balsamic sauce.

How to Add Flavour Without Using Too Much Sugar or Fat:

Use aromatic bottles of vinegar, citrus juices, herbs, and spices to lift the flavor of your side dishes without relying on heavy fats or sugars.

To add depth and complexity to your recipes, try experimenting with spices like cumin, paprika, or ginger, as well as aromatic herbs like basil, cilantro, or dill.

To add brightness and acidity, use citrus zest, lemon juice, or balsamic vinegar. This will improve the overall flavor profile of your side dishes without sacrificing nutrition.

Techniques for Reducing the Portion of Side Dishes:

Portion control is crucial, especially for those who are managing gastroparesis, even though side dishes are an integral part of a balanced meal.

To keep things in proportion and avoid overindulging, try to consume half of your plate with non-starchy veggies, 1/4 with a lean protein source, and 1/4 with a starchy or grain-based side dish.

Pay attention to your body's signals of hunger and fullness, and use smaller bowls or plates to help you control portion sizes.

Creating delicious side dishes that both suit your palate and your dietary requirements is essential to managing your gastroparesis effectively. You can prepare a variety of side dishes that promote your health and well-being by experimenting with gentle cooking methods, adding nutrient-rich ingredients, and using flavor-enhancing approaches.

Desserts and Sweet Treats:

Desserts and sweets are frequently thought of as decadent delights, but they can be problematic for people with gastroparesis because of their potential to worsen symptoms like bloating, nausea, and pain.

Desserts can be both filling and easy on the stomach, though, if careful preparation and inventive preparation are used.

Desserts That Are Both Rich and Nutritious:

Sweet treats don't always have to be associated with bad decisions. Actually, there are a lot of solutions that can nourish and support general health in addition to satisfying a sweet taste. It is crucial for people with gastroparesis to choose desserts high in fiber, vitamins, and minerals. Desserts made with fruits, whole grains, nuts, and seeds can fulfill cravings and support a healthy diet at the same time.

Recipes for sugarless desserts:

For those who are managing gastroparesis, cutting back on sugar is usually advised because high-sugar foods can exacerbate symptoms and cause blood sugar swings. Recipes for low-sugar desserts emphasize the use of naturally sweet ingredients such as fruits and dried fruits, together with alternative sweeteners like erythritol, stevia, and monk fruit. These desserts are excellent for those with diabetes and gastroparesis since they have a sweet taste without quickly raising blood sugar levels.

Desserts made with fruit for a naturally sweet taste:

Fruits can make a delectable complement to sweets without the need for additional sugar because they are inherently sweet. Fruit-based desserts use the inherent sweetness of fruits such as mangoes, pears, apples, and berries to make tasty, pleasantly acidic treats. Fruits are a cool, healthy substitute for conventional desserts, whether they are eaten raw, cooked, or mixed into smoothies or sorbets.

Advice on how to sate desires without sacrificing your health objectives:

While following dietary limitations can make it difficult to control urges, it is possible to do so in a way that supports your health objectives by using mindful tactics. Nuts, spices, and dark chocolate are examples of flavor- and texture-rich ingredients that can improve dessert delight without adding too much sugar or fat. Cravings can also be sated with smaller servings by emphasizing the sensory aspects of eating, such as enjoying flavors and textures.

Techniques for regulating dessert portion sizes:

Desserts should be enjoyed in moderation, especially for those who are managing gastroparesis. Meals should be smaller and more often in order to avoid overfeeding the stomach and reduce discomfort. Desserts with portion controls, such as little fruit parfaits, single-serving custards, or mini cupcakes, let you indulge without overtaxing your digestive tract. Additionally, mindful eating practices can improve enjoyment and support digestive comfort. These practices include chewing gently and enjoying every bite.

Innovative methods to add antioxidants to sweets:

Adding antioxidants to sweet foods can have additional health benefits since they help shield the body from harm caused by free radicals. Desserts can be made more antioxidant-rich by creatively using foods like dark chocolate, berries, nuts, and spices like cloves and cinnamon. These components raise antioxidant levels, which promote general health and well-being, in addition to improving the taste and texture of desserts. Antioxidant-rich sweets that are both delicious and healthful can be made by experimenting with different mixes and recipes.

Smoothies and Beverages:

Smoothies and drinks are important dietary choices for controlling gastroparesis since they are easy on the stomach and supply vital nutrients. Including hydrated and nutrient-dense foods can aid with symptom relief and promote general health.

CHAPTER SEVEN

Ideas for Refreshing and Hydrating Drinks: For those who have gastroparesis, staying hydrated is crucial since dehydration can make symptoms like weariness and nausea worse. Fruit-infused water, such as that made with cucumber, lemon, or berries, is a hydrating beverage option that tastes good without adding extra sugar. Another great option is coconut water, which is hydration-rich and replaces electrolytes.

Smoothie Recipes Packed with Nutrients: Smoothies are a great method to get enough nutrients without overtaxing the digestive system. Smoothies can be made more stomach-friendly by using easily digested ingredients like cooked veggies, ripe bananas, and nut butter. Maintaining energy levels and promoting muscular function can also be achieved by including protein sources, such as Greek yogurt or protein powder.

Components:

One ripe banana

1/2 cup of sweet potatoes, cooked

One spoonful of butter made of almonds

Half a cup of spinach

1/2 cup almond milk (or your preferred non-dairy milk)

Ice cubes, if desired

Guidelines:

Put everything into a blender.

Blend till creamy and smooth.

If you want the texture to be colder, add ice cubes.

After pouring into a glass, savor!

Choices of Herbal Teas to Help with Digestion:

Herbal teas can help people with gastroparesis feel better by improving digestion and lowering nausea. Due to its reputation for reducing bloating and stomach symptoms, peppermint tea is a great option for people who are uncomfortable. Another well-liked choice is ginger tea, which can ease nausea and settle the stomach.

The Value of Maintaining Hydration

Maintaining general health and controlling the symptoms of gastroparesis depend on enough water. Dehydration can worsen symptoms like exhaustion, constipation, and lightheadedness, so it's critical to consume enough fluids throughout the day. Make it a point to consume eight glasses of water or more each day, and think about including items high in hydration, including fruits and vegetables, in your diet.

Suggestions for Cutting Back on Sugar-Coated Drinks:

Drinks with high sugar content might exacerbate the symptoms of gastroparesis by delaying digestion and elevating blood sugar levels. Use unsweetened beverages instead of sugary ones, including water, herbal tea, or water that has been infused with fresh fruit and herbs. If you're in want of something sweet, try utilizing natural sweeteners like honey or maple syrup sparingly.

Innovative Methods for Naturally Flavouring Water:

Naturally flavored water can add flavor and appeal to the act of staying hydrated. Play around with different fruit, vegetable, and herb combinations to make infused water options that are delightful. Cucumber and mint, lemon and basil, or orange and ginger are a few delectable pairings. Furthermore, enjoying flavored water on the go can be made simple by using a pitcher or bottle with a built-in fruit infusion.

People can improve their general health and digestive health while enjoying delicious and nutritional options by adding these smoothie and beverage ideas to a cookbook for managing gastroparesis.

Social Events and Eating Out:

Being a person with gastroparesis can make navigating restaurants and social gatherings particularly difficult, but with a little planning and knowledge, you can still enjoy social events without sacrificing your health objectives.

Investigate Restaurants in Advance:

Check out menu possibilities at restaurants by calling them ahead of time or doing an internet search before you go. These days, a lot of restaurants provide their menus, complete with nutritional data, online, so you can plan ahead.

Select Restaurants with Flexible Menus: Choose eateries that have dishes that can be customized or that offer a range of selections that can accommodate your dietary requirements. Asian culinary traditions, such as Thai and Japanese, frequently feature meals that are easily adaptable to meet dietary requirements.

Communicate Clearly with Servers: Don't be afraid to let your server know about any dietary limitations you may have when placing an order. Briefly and courteously describe your condition, and inquire about the preparation of the dishes. The majority of eateries are adaptable and ready to change to suit your requirements.

Be Ready to Adjust Meals: **Occasionally, even with good communication, you can discover that some of the menu alternatives don't fully meet your needs. In these situations, don't be afraid to request adjustments, such as changing the cooking process or eliminating specific ingredients.**

Emphasis on Easy Preparations: **Choose foods that are easily cooked, like grilled or steamed foods, as these are typically less taxing on the stomach and less likely to aggravate symptoms of gastroparesis.**

Control Your Portion: **If you have gastroparesis, in particular, restaurant portions are frequently larger than what you may require. To prevent overindulging, think about splitting a meal with a dining partner or asking for a half serving.**

How to Effectively Communicate Your Dietary Needs:

Be Particular and Clear: Try to be as particular and clear as you can when expressing your dietary requirements. Describe your illness and any special dietary needs you may have because of your gastroparesis, such as avoiding fatty or high-fiber meals.

Employ Positive Language: Instead of focusing on what you cannot consume, frame your dietary requirements in a positive perspective. By doing this, miscommunications can be avoided and it will be simpler for others to meet your demands.

Offer Suggestions: Don't be afraid to ask your waitress for recommendations or other selections if you have questions regarding the menu. They might be able to suggest foods that fit your dietary requirements.

Express Your Gratitude: Thank the restaurant personnel for whatever accomodations they may have made. Saying "thank you" is a small but effective approach to establishing a good rapport with restaurant staff.

Techniques for Handling Social Events Without Sacrificing Health Objectives:

Make a Plan: Before attending a social event, discuss your dietary requirements with the host. Make sure there is at least one food that is suitable for people with gastroparesis by offering to bring one that you can eat and share with others.

Eat Before You Go: You might want to have a quick supper or snack before you leave the house if you're not sure what food options are available. This may lessen the need to eat things that could aggravate the symptoms of gastroparesis and help prevent hunger.

Emphasis on Socialising: Place more emphasis on mingling and enjoying each other's company at social gatherings than on the cuisine. Talk to others, take part in events, or offer assistance with non-food-related chores.

Bring Your Own Snacks: If you're going to an event where food will be provided, think about bringing light meals or snacks that are suitable for someone with gastroparesis. In the event that your options for food are restricted, this guarantees you have something safe to consume.

CHAPTER EIGHT
Making Nutritious Decisions When Dining Out

Stick to Simple, Whole Foods: When dining out, give preference to simple, digestible foods that are whole. Lean proteins, cooked veggies, and whole grains may be examples of this. Steer clear of processed or high-fat foods since these may make your gastroparesis symptoms worse.

Remain Hydrated: Controlling the symptoms of gastroparesis requires maintaining adequate hydration. When dining out, choose water or other non-carbonated, non-caffeinated beverages instead of alcohol, which can exacerbate symptoms.

Listen to Your Body: Observe how eating certain foods affects your mood and modify your diet accordingly. If particular foods seem to cause symptoms on a regular basis, steer clear of them going forward, even if they are served when dining out.

Be Aware of Portion Sizes: When dining out, watch your portion sizes to prevent overindulging and undue stress on your digestive system. If servings are overly large, ask for a to-go container so you can preserve leftovers for another time.

Ideas for Organising Events That Are Gastroparesis-Friendly:

If you're throwing a party and you are aware of someone's dietary needs, such as gastroparesis, get in touch with them ahead of time to make sure appropriate

Serve a Range of Foods: Serve a range of foods that satisfy various nutritional requirements, such as those with low fat, high fiber content, and spicy components.

Dishes should have clear labels that list any allergies or dietary requirements.

Add Options That Are Gastroparesis-Friendly: Include items on your menu that are suitable for people with gastroparesis, such as simple carbs, lean proteins, and well-cooked vegetables. Take into account dishes that are simple to adapt to meet particular dietary requirements.

Urge Guests to Bring food: Let them know if they have any dietary restrictions and ask them to bring food to share. This lessens the workload for the host and guarantees a wide variety of foods.

Establish a Comfortable Ambience: Make sure there is enough seating for everyone and foster a laid-back, cozy environment for your visitors. Pay attention to each other's company instead of just the meal.

These techniques can help people with gastroparesis navigate social situations and eat out more easily and joyfully, as well as their friends and family. In order to ensure that everyone can fully participate in social activities while prioritizing health and well-being, communication, preparation, and flexibility are essential.

Upkeep and Extended Success:

The management of gastroparesis is a continuous process that calls for commitment and tenacity. Successful long-term management of gastroparesis requires careful maintenance. To reduce symptoms and improve general well-being, this entails making durable dietary and lifestyle adjustments and following medical advice.

Maintaining Your Progress in Gastroparesis Management

Maintaining your gastroparesis treatment plan requires perseverance, forbearance, and constancy. To effectively manage symptoms, you must prioritize self-care activities and develop routines that support your health goals. This could involve organizing meals, controlling medications, practicing stress management, and routinely checking symptoms.

The significance of routine check-ins with medical professionals

Keeping in close contact with medical professionals is essential for managing gastroparesis.

These consultations enable the tracking of symptoms, assessment of the efficacy of treatment, and necessary modifications to the management plan. Healthcare professionals can provide helpful advice, recommend dietary changes, write prescriptions for drugs, and offer support for any issues or difficulties encountered during the management process.

Techniques for maintaining accountability and motivation

Maintaining motivation and accountability is critical to the long-term management of gastroparesis. Motivation can be sustained by establishing reasonable goals, monitoring development, and acknowledging successes. Involving loved ones in your journey, joining support groups, and asking medical professionals for assistance can also offer accountability and encouragement.

Advice for overcoming obstacles along the route:

Managing gastroparesis may present some challenges, but there are ways to get around them. Effective remedies can be found by keeping a symptom diary, recognizing triggers, and experimenting with alternative dietary approaches. It's also critical to be transparent with healthcare professionals about any challenges you face in order to get the help and direction you need.

Including exercise to promote general well-being:

Being physically active is essential for maintaining general health, which includes controlling the symptoms of gastroparesis. While some people may find that intense exercise makes their symptoms worse, milder exercises like swimming, yoga, or walking might be helpful. Frequent exercise enhances mood, lowers stress levels, and helps with digestion, all of which contribute to a higher quality of life.

Rejoicing your accomplishments and maintaining an optimistic outlook:
Acknowledging accomplishments, regardless of their magnitude, is crucial for preserving

drive and optimism during the gastroparesis treatment process. Acknowledging accomplishments, conquering obstacles, and recognizing progress can strengthen positive behaviors and increase self-esteem. Embracing thankfulness, maintaining an optimistic outlook, and concentrating on your controllables will help you weather the ups and downs of gastroparesis management with fortitude and hope.

The meals and meal plans shown below are ones that are intended for a patient with gastroparesis and promote healthy living.

Recipes:

Oatmeal Banana Smoothie:

To make a smooth breakfast, blend together 1/2 cup cooked oats, 1/2 cup plain Greek yogurt, and a pinch of cinnamon with one ripe banana.

Lunch:

Dinner:

Chicken with Mashed Sweet Potatoes:

Morning meal:

For lunch, have 1/2 cup of cooked chicken breast that has been shredded on top of mashed sweet potatoes.

Dinner:

Scrambled eggs and spinach:

For breakfast, scramble two eggs with low-fat cheese and sautéed spinach.

Lunch:

Dinner:

Carrot Soup with Ginger:

Morning meal:

Lunch: Refresh yourself with a cup of low-sodium broth, pureed cooked carrots, and ginger.

Dinner:

Salmon baked with quinoa:

Morning meal:

Lunch:

Supper: Present a baked salmon fillet accompanied by steaming green beans and a dish of fluffy quinoa.

Pancakes and Fried Rice:

Morning meal:

Lunch: Savour a warm bowl of turkey and rice congee, which is made with white rice, low-sodium broth, and shredded turkey breast.

Dinner:

Pancakes with cottage cheese:

For breakfast, savor fluffy pancakes cooked with eggs, blended cottage cheese, and a touch of vanilla flavor.

Lunch:

Dinner:

Soup with Roasted Butternut Squash:

Morning meal:

Lunch: Enjoy a bowl of roasted butternut squash soup with a dollop of Greek yogurt and a hint of nutmeg.

Dinner:

Stir-fried Tofu with Vegetables:

Morning meal:

For lunch, try stir-frying cubed tofu with a rainbow of vibrant veggies, including broccoli,

Dinner:

Apples Baked with Cinnamon:

Morning meal:

Lunch:

Dinner: For a pleasant and calming way to round off the day, treat yourself to a baked apple dusted with cinnamon.

30-Day Meal Plan:

Day 1–10:

Banana muesli smoothie for breakfast

Lunch is chicken with mashed sweet potatoes.

Dinner is spinach and egg scramble.

Day 11–20:

Ginger Carrot Soup for Breakfast

Quinoa with Baked Salmon for Lunch

Dinner is rice congee and turkey.

Day 21–30:

Pancakes with cottage cheese for breakfast

Roasted Butternut Squash Soup for lunch

Vegetable Stir-Fry with Tofu for Dinner

You are welcome to modify serving sizes and meal schedules in accordance with personal tastes and dietary requirements. Furthermore, keep in mind that before making any big dietary adjustments, particularly for the treatment of a condition like gastroparesis, you should speak with a medical professional or certified dietitian.

In summary

Finally, I hope that my cookbook will be a helpful resource for anyone attempting to manage their gastroparesis through diet, acting as a ray of hope. A sophisticated eating strategy that emphasizes simple digestion, mild ingredients, and careful amount control is necessary for those with gastroparesis. We've covered a wide range of recipes and cooking techniques on these pages, all of which are tailored to meet your preferences.

But keep in mind that this cookbook is only the start. Your experience with gastroparesis is distinct, and as time goes on, your dietary requirements may change. I urge you to stay involved with your healthcare team, pay attention to your body's cues, and keep an open mind about what might be the greatest option for you as you proceed down this path.

Above all, I hope that this book will serve as a source of delicious nourishment, empowerment, and inspiration for you as you pursue wellness. Let's embrace every meal as a chance to grow, one bite at a time.

THE END

www.ingramcontent.com/pod-product-compliance
Lightning Source LLC
Chambersburg PA
CBHW052332220526
45472CB00001B/387